Pray.Ea
My Journey Through
Weight Loss

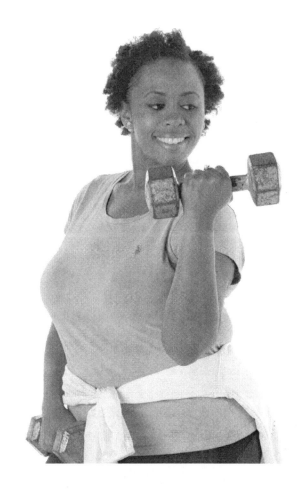

By Meagan Pinkney

DEDICATION

This book is dedicated to everyone that needs encouragement
along their weight loss journey.

CONTENTS

Acknowledgments   vii

Introduction   viii

Chapter One ~The Situation   1

Chapter Two ~ The Weight Is Over   8

Reflection   43

Principles for a Productive   46

Weight Loss Journey

Before Pictures   54

After Pictures   55

Transition Pictures   56

ACKNOWLEDGMENTS

I would first like to thank God the Father, God the Son and God the Holy Spirit for choosing me to experience this amazing journey! I would also like to acknowledge my trainer Dominique, founder of Built2Last and my family and friends for the encouragement and for putting up with me during my moments.

Thank you!

INTRODUCTION

In today's society, everyone wants to know how to lose weight instantly. Some recommendations are to explore those celebrity and military diets or just simply not eating. To be honest, if this could be done everyone would do it...right? Being conscious of our weight or waistline is something that a majority of people can relate to. According to the Centers for Disease Control and Prevention (CDC), more than one-third (34.9% or 78.6 million) of U.S. adults are obese. I can only speak for myself that I do not want to be included in that 34.9%, but in reality I was stuck there for several years of my young life until something changed! In this book, I will share my personal testimony of my supernatural weight loss journey. My journey, although quite unique, will encourage you and hopefully kick-start your own personal weight loss journey and relationship with the Holy Spirit. Whether we realize it or not the excess weight that we are physically carrying around is a huge hindrance to our productiveness in life. Once we can develop a healthy balance of praying, eating and lifting then our journey can begin.

—

God Bless

CHAPTER ONE ~ THE SITUATION

As a young child growing up in Southern Louisiana, food was my friend. My favorite foods were bread and rice and I just had to have rice with just about every meal that I ate. Eating those in excess was probably not the best thing to do. But when you're a child you really don't know. Now, I wasn't necessarily overweight growing up, but if you continue in that particular lifestyle it catches up with you really quickly. Luckily, by the time I entered into high school I had an interest in playing on the girl's basketball team, which I made my freshmen year. I was also on the track and field team for my high school my freshmen year. My time on these teams allowed me to lower my high blood pressure, become physically active and lose some weight. I remember being in high school and a guy on the boy's basketball team told a friend of mine that, "Meagan would be really pretty if she just lost more weight". Wow, thanks for the encouraging words! I never considered myself to be ugly or unattractive but the excess weight definitely affected my self-esteem and confidence around other people (especially the opposite sex). I was tired of being the "big" one in the group. I also remember a guy from high school that I liked who told his cousin that he liked me too, but he didn't want to date me. Who does that?! I wasn't informed if his decision was due to my weight or not but in my young mind this added fuel to my self-esteem issues. It was also brought to me that I was jealous of my twin sister because she was much thinner than I was. Really?! You name it; I've probably heard it. I try not to let other people's opinions affect negatively my way of thinking; especially about myself. However, I am human and it does hurt sometimes. As a Christian, the enemy in our life tries every tactic and scheme to keep you low and down and focused on things that don't even matter. I thank God that He was watching over me even then because only He knows what could have happened if I took to heart those negative comments towards me at that young age. One thing I can say is that I never set my goals in life such as weight loss to please other people- I feel that those goals will always be short lived.

During my high school years, I was able to maintain my smaller weight and entered into college healthier than ever. However, because I didn't continue my physical activity and semi-healthy lifestyle throughout college guess what?? The weight came back and since my physical activity was taken away and a new phase of my life was starting, maintaining my weight was not on the top of my to-do list. Over the next four years of college, I found that my weight slowly crept back into my life. But with all of the excitement of graduating from college, I did not even realize it. How could that be? It's really easy especially when there was no physical activity taking place and my eating lifestyle was under no control. Before I knew it I was well over 200 pounds. Being that I am only 5'5" this makes me extremely obese. From a fitness test that I once took at a gym, it was discovered that my bones were heavy (dense) which is a good thing however I was still well over 200 pounds!!

By this stage of my life, I began to wonder if the food was really the issue? Yes, of course, the food entering my body causes the pounds to increase, but what was causing me to eat in this manner? Was I stressing due to school issues? No, I had graduated from high school and college with honors. Was I concerned about obtaining a job after college? No, I had obtained a full-time job with a great company even before I had graduated from college. Well, what could it be? This is the question that most people that are struggling with their weight ask themselves at least once in their lives. The answer varies with each individual but could range from low self-esteem, emotional challenges or even lifestyle. I'll say all of the above for me.

After graduating from college, I made serious efforts to reintroduce exercise back into my life. Good news...I actually lost weight but, unfortunately, it was short-lived....again! Every time that my schedule would change, exercise was the first activity that was cut from my schedule. If you could imagine this type of behavior won't result in lifelong weight loss. At this point, I had finally made up my mind and decided that it was time for a change.

Individuals ask me now, Meagan, did you go on a diet? No, I didn't. I simply changed my lifestyle. Some may ask, what's the big deal with these lifestyle changes? Well, eating fried chicken every day or hamburgers every day isn't wise. The average person knows that but yet we still do it. To start off my weight loss journey, I made a decision to not live to eat but instead eat to live. The Word of God says in Matthew 4:4,

"Jesus answered, "It is written: 'Man shall not live on bread

alone, but on every word that comes from the mouth of God.'"

　

During my weight loss journey, I truly wanted to write

down in a book my experience so that it will be an

encouragement to those individuals looking to change their

lifestyle and yet get closer to God in the process.

CHAPTER TWO ~ THE WEIGHT IS OVER

In my 28 years of being on this Earth, I began to grow tired of the WEIGHT that I was. As a result, I had a talk with my Heavenly Father about my concerns. Now this talk wasn't necessarily a full-blown prayer but a simple conversation one would have with a close friend. The setting was in Tulsa, Oklahoma in my one bedroom apartment. I had recently moved back to Tulsa, OK with my job but all on assignment for the Lord. I sat down one day in December 2013 and made known my request. The New Year was quickly approaching and naturally the number one New Year's resolution for most people is to lose weight. This was indeed my resolution for the upcoming year but I was very specific in my asking and resolution goals. My conversation and request went something like the following:

"Lord, I really want to lose weight. I not only want to lose weight, but I want to keep it off for life! I would like to be a size 6. When I get married and my husband and I begin to have children, I would like the ability to breastfeed all of my children and naturally go right back down to my size 6."

After my conversation with God, nothing huge happened. The weight didn't instantly fall off my body nor did I feel any different. One thing that I do know is that my request was genuine and from a pure place in my heart. My motives for weight loss were certainly not to gain the attention from men or impress anyone. I simply knew that my size wasn't God's plan for my life and it wasn't pleasing Him. I knew in my heart that whatever my purpose was for being on this Earth, the weight had to leave. My request to God was made in faith and without WORKS faith is dead (James 2:20). My works began by simply joining a gym and thankfully there was a Gold's gym very close to my apartment. One Saturday morning I walked into Gold's gym inquiring about their membership and application process. As I sat at the desk of the training specialist, he looked at me and asked me one simple question- "What is my goal for joining the gym?" I answered, "I want to lose weight". Naturally his next question was, "How much weight?" I answered with no hesitation, "50 pounds". Before then, I had never really thought about the actual number of pounds I wanted to lose I just knew that I wanted to lose weight.

HINT When making your weight loss goals be as specific as possible. Also make reachable goals in reachable timeframes (i.e., I want to lose 20 pounds in 3 months)

At this time, I was a little over the 250-pound mark and the goal to lose 50 pounds was definitely a stretch for me. As previously stated, I had lost weight before but nowhere near 50 pounds. I would say 20 pounds was my top weight loss amount up until that point. Did I truly believe that I could lose 50 pounds? Yes, I was determined! But this time, was different from the previous attempts. This attempt had a purpose! I didn't approach this weight loss journey haphazardly; I was intentional and very focused. I was so focused during this journey that the

Holy Spirit had to call me on the rug at times in His loving way

of course. I will discuss that situation shortly.

Back to my conversation with the training specialist, he

took note of my weight loss goal and suggested that I obtain a

personal trainer for encouragement, accountability, and targeted

weight loss. I would personally consider myself to be a self-

motivated individual, but I figured if I wanted something I never

had I must do something that I have never done before.

Personal trainer it was! Oh wait, how much is a personal trainer,

I asked him. It was around $60/per session, which is typically

one hour. Well, in that case, I agreed to have one personal

training session every two weeks starting off to see how it goes.

The other days would be focused on a rotation between the

machines and the personal weights. One of the BEST perks at

this gym was the theater! I had never seen a gym with a movie theater room with various exercise machines in it. You can watch your favorite movies while burning serious calories. I love to watch movies, therefore, this room became one of my favorite rooms (anything helps!). God is good!

As discussed, the training specialist scheduled my first personal training session right off the bat. I specifically requested a female trainer and my request was granted. I truly thank God for her because she helped me tremendously to kick-start this weight loss journey. By January 2014, I was an active member at a gym with a personal trainer. My New Year's request to God was starting off great! To make things even sweeter my Pastor announced that our church was going on a Daniel's fast starting the second week in January. I was familiar with this fast and knew no meats or sweets were allowed to be eaten for 21 days. The combination of working out and being in a time of consecration made my focus and weight loss journey accelerate. By the end of the 21 days of fasting and working out, I lost around 10 pounds! This was extremely encouraging and motivating. As I continued on my journey my personal trainer gave me some terrible news- she was quitting her personal trainer position at the gym! What?! Right when things seem to be working out so great this happens. She informed me that they had already hired her replacement and I would meet her at my next training session. I wasn't happy and really wasn't interested in training with another individual. I was comfortable with her, but at that time I didn't realize that God was rewarding my efforts and taking me to the next level in my journey. I thought to myself if I didn't like this new trainer right off the bat my next training session would be my last training session with a personal trainer.

Here we go! I entered the gym 10-15 minutes before my training session started with my new trainer. I walked over to the stretching center and saw a face I had never seen before at the stretching center. I believe we started a small conversation and from our conversation I discovered something very interesting and hilarious. This nice lady was my new trainer! Praise God..lol. We both laughed and began our workout session. Within minutes of the workout session, I quickly noticed that her style of a workout was very different from my previous trainer. She was down to business and she didn't play! I loved it! It was now March 2014 and I noticed that my clothes were getting too big. At least 3 days a week I would make my way to the gym to stay active and stay focused on my goal. Personally, I only checked my weight on the scale at the gym maybe once a month. This may sound crazy to some people, but your actual weight number fluctuates so much and is dependent on other factors, I have never really obsessed about my weight number. For my current goal, I truly desired to be a size 6... for life!

HINT When you're starting your weight loss journey, make sure to stay focused on developing your workout routine and sticking to it versus checking the scale every day.

One Saturday during my training session with my new trainer I was informed of more terrible news. She, too, was quitting her personal trainer position at the gym! Really?! This isn't funny anymore. My trainer tells me that she started her own workout company and it's a boot camp style workout. Her daily workouts are in the evenings for only $60 a month! Wow! I told her wherever you go I'm going. I kept my gym membership for a little while after her leaving but it was later canceled.

Her workouts were like nothing I had ever experienced since my high school basketball conditioning days ten years ago. I was really excited about this new challenge. Just to give you an idea of the type of workout we were doing, we started working out at a high school football field running up and down the bleachers (the entire length of the field, down and back) just for our WARMUPS! I also liked this boot camp style workout because it wasn't just me working out. It was a group of people out there with a common goal- weight loss. Our workouts were different every week and intensified as my strength began to increase. To be transparent, there were some exercises that we were to do on the football field that I couldn't do physically because of my weight. I literally wasn't able to hold my own body weight with my arms. I told my trainer one day I'll be able to perform that exercise with no problem. And that "one-day" actually came! Maybe a month later my trainer challenged me to perform that same exercise and I performed it with no problem!

HINT One of the true signs of success during your weight loss journey is your PROGRESS! Make sure to take note of these "progress moments."

It is now May 2014 and I'm feeling great! I haven't reached my weight loss goal yet but progress is being made for sure plus I was enjoying the journey. By this point, I hope that you've been encouraged and are ready to start or restart your weight loss journey with me. I could end this book now and go on with my life, however, something amazing happened in my life around this time that I MUST share. God answered my

prayer! Do you remember when I mentioned earlier in my story

that I had a conversation with God (prayer) regarding my weight

loss journey? And the specific things that I desired? In case you

don't remember my conversation mentioned I think it bears

repeating. My request went something like the following:

"Lord, I really want to lose weight. I not only want to

lose weight, but I want to keep it off for life! I would like to be a

size 6. When I get married and my husband and I begin to have

children, I would like the ability to breastfeed all of my children

and naturally go right back down to my size 6."

Well, I was informed about a prayer conference that was

to take place in early May and I simply wanted to serve at the event. The Pastors that were hosting the prayer conference attended my church, but I had never met them personally. In fact, I had never heard about a prayer conference in my life. Is it just a conference talking about prayer? I had no idea, but I genuinely wanted to serve. At this point, you're probably wondering why I'm including information about my serving at this prayer conference? That's a very good question and you'll see why as you keep reading on. The conference was scheduled to be four days long and I requested to be on the registration team. On the first day of the conference, I was walking into the hotel conference building when I ran into some folks from my church and particularly one lady I had met recently at our bible study. We all walked in together and received our serving assignments for the conference. I was excited all day long about serving on the registration team and to my amazement the positions on the registration team were already taken. I wasn't too happy but I quickly remembered I am there to serve, period.

I asked the volunteer leader what other areas were there that needed filling. She said that they needed more ushers to welcome the individuals into the hotel and direct them to the conference room. I agreed to be an usher and so did the lady that I walked in with from church. I reintroduced myself to her as we walked to our assigned post. We are both friendly people so our time serving together was very enjoyable. In between welcoming the guest to the conference we began to chat and learn more about each other. She is definitely a talker so I just let her talk and I interjected as needed. I truly didn't feel led to share a lot about myself so I just listened. Once our serving assignment was complete we both entered the conference for an amazing time. I drove home after the conference and my serving friend was on my mind, however, we never exchanged numbers. I just hoped that she'd be serving at the conference for the second night.

The second night came and I was in the position to serve as an usher to welcome the guest to the conference and my friend was nowhere to be found. Moments later she arrived! She walked up to me and we greeted each other and she said I have to share with you what the Holy Spirit told me last night during the prayer conference. I said okay, I'm excited and I can't wait to hear what the Lord said about you. Then she said something that caught me off guard. She said, no He didn't speak to me about me but you, Meagan. Really? Now I'm really listening! She began to speak the exact words that were spoken from my heart during my conversation with God! No, really, word for word!

She said....

"Meagan, God is going to take your weight away for His glory. You will be around a size 6 and once you get married and start having children God will allow you to breastfeed your children and go right back down to a size 6. Your weight loss will be God putting His super on your natural efforts. He is simply displaying the beauty that He's created on the inside of you and showing it outwardly. This is for your future- ministry and marriage. She then began to pray over me and spoke directly to my fat cells and commanded them to leave. Finally, she gave me some instructions. She said the Lord wants you to go on a Daniel's Fast for 21 days and pray and focus on weight loss and at the end of the fast sow a seed into good ground to seal the deal."

I couldn't do anything but lift my hands and receive what the Holy Spirit was telling me and confirming that He had indeed heard my prayer. Some may be thinking well maybe Meagan told a close friend her desire and prayer in an effort to touch and agree and it made its way to this lady. I'm here to tell you I did not tell one person about my desire or prayer. I honestly didn't feel it necessary to share with even my close friends because my desire was communicated out of my intimate time with the Lord. The scripture comes to mind about the Samaritan woman at the well. After she spoke with Jesus and He told her about her life she left Him and went into town telling everyone to come see a man who told her everything she did.

"The woman left her water jar beside the well and ran back to the village, telling everyone, "Come and see a man who told me everything I ever did! Could he possibly be the Messiah?" So the people came streaming from the village to see him." John 4:28-30

NLT

This is how I truly felt! I was shocked, surprised, excited and ready all at the same time. From that moment on, my life took a drastic change. We finished serving at the prayer conference and it was awesome! The conference ended on a Sunday and that Monday I started my Daniel's Fast. More fruits, veggies and lots of water! I didn't know how this journey would look or feel but I was one determined and motivated young lady. I was so determined and convinced that I was going to be a size 6 and remain my size 6 forever, I started to "sow" my clothes into the lives of individuals in my church. I would literally ask women around my size if they needed any clothes...free of charge. I started giving away bags full of clothes every week to various people. It got so serious to people that they would boldly walk up to me after church on any given Sunday and look at the clothes tag on my neck collar and say, "I want this one". It was crazy! By the way, I'm not referring to clothes that I couldn't fit any longer, I was strictly walking by faith and releasing my past size and making room for my future size. As my giving increased, my receiving increased as well. I received a call from a friend in town saying that the Holy Spirit instructed her to purchase a nice dress for me in my smaller size! I received several pairs of nice high heel shoes from another young lady from church. I also received a large box full of clothes from someone I don't even know! Some of the items that I received I kept for myself but some of the items I sowed into the lives of other ladies as the Holy Spirit instructed me to. I was getting used to receiving these great new clothes that I almost forgot that it's better to give than to receive.

"And I have been a constant example of how you can help those in need by working hard. You should remember the words of the Lord Jesus: 'It is more blessed to give than to receive.'" Acts

20:35 NLT

Most of the time I just kept the clothes and shoes that I knew that I was to sow that I received from other people in the truck of my car and gave as led. I had literally turned into a distribution center for the Kingdom of God! Without planning, I began collecting clothes and shoes from individuals around town for my recently started non-profit organization, The Joseph Foundation. The mission of the Joseph Foundation is to obtain and distribute personal items such as but not limited to clothes, shoes, water and food donated by the general public or purchased for the distribution of those in need across the World. With no flyer designed or posted, I was able to collect several bags of clothes for the organization that were placed in my personal climate controlled storage. One day while visiting my storage to pay my monthly bill, I heard that small still voice say, "Ask them how much does it cost to rent a small storage just for the organization". A little hesitate, I turned my car around and went back to the storage office and asked the question just as I heard it. To my surprise, I was able to get a student discount on my personal storage and get a small storage for the organization with the student discount as well! I tell you, it really does benefit us when we obey the instructions of the Holy Spirit whether they make sense at the time or not. Also, the lady that worked at the storage inquired about my organization and was more than excited to donate several bags of her clothes as well!! Once I received the organization's storage, clothes and shoes came from everywhere! For example, a co-worker of mine was relocating back to Mexico for work and he was cleaning out his personal things in his apartment and was looking to give certain things away. He approached me one day at work saying that he wanted to give me several boxes of his new clothes because he trusted me and knew that I would know what to do with the clothes! No one at my job knew anything about The Joseph Foundation, therefore, I KNEW this was a confirmation from the Holy Spirit that He was indeed in this movement. I quickly informed my co-worker about my organization and he was just as shocked as I was about this entire situation. The beautiful thing about this is that the individual wasn't a Christian but after this connection he was more comfortable with me and warmed up to Christianity. He even accepted my invitation to visit my church one Sunday morning and he not only attended and enjoyed himself, he even invited a friend of his!

One step of faith to purchase the storage unit opened the floodgates of Heaven for the organization to receive extreme overflow. In no time that small storage was filled to capacity and a much larger storage was rented for the organization. In 2015, The Joseph Foundation was able to bless several families in the North Tulsa community. We also donated several items to churches needing clothes for distribution, an Evangelism Ministry for the homeless, a Prison Ministry for women and planted a financial seed to assist a daily feeding program for orphans and Aids patients in Durban, South Africa! Needless to say, the momentum that kick-started my efforts at The Joseph Foundation was all started from me sowing my personal clothes by faith.

If you or someone you know may be interested in donating to The Joseph Foundation please contact us by the information below:

www.meaganpinkney.com

539-302-3848

thejosephfoundations@gmail.com

Moving back to my weight loss journey, it is now the end of my God instructed Daniel's Fast. I've lost more weight and was very excited about my journey. I was also really enjoying my boot camp workouts. But I needed to sow my seed as instructed, but to whom? I was thinking that the person the Holy Spirit wanted me to sow the seed to was the young lady that the Holy Spirit used to minister to me. After much prayer I got it! I was to sow the seed into the life of my trainer. You may be wondering why I took the time to pray for the person to sow the seed into? First, this was an important matter for me and I needed to have the right person. Secondly, not all ground is good ground to sow into, therefore, I needed the wisdom and direction from the Holy Spirit. The last day of the fast I asked the Holy Spirit what was the amount to be sown. A financial figure popped into my head and I asked for confirmation before I left for the workout. I felt the Holy Spirit speak to my heart, this is the amount and this is the person. That word was settled in my spirit and I was off to workout! I texted my trainer earlier that day to bring her Square to take my payment even though it wasn't my pay week, I was glad that she didn't question my request. But I guess who would if you're giving them money! The workout was great and I acted as usual without any suggestion of the situation. After the workout was over my trainer and I walked over to our cars to make the payment. As she reached for the Square device, I began to explain the situation. I shared with her my prayer to the Lord about my weight loss, my confirmation, and clear instructions from the

Holy Spirit at the Prayer Conference and my need to sow a seed. I informed her that she was the person I was to sow the seed into and the amount I had in my heart was the right amount. All that was great but the most touching part of my communication with my trainer were the tears that were flowing from her eyes. The tears were certainly not about the money because although I told her about the seed that was to be sown that day I never mentioned to her the dollar amount. When I saw her tears, it let me know that the Holy Spirit had touched her heart during our conversation about my testimony in the making. Wow! I finally reached for the Square device and typed in my seed amount of $500 and swiped my card and signed to complete the transaction. I handed her the Square back and told her the amount and more tears flowed. She began to tell me that right before she arrived at the workout that day she went to visit her grandmother's house to ask her for $20 for gas money because she only had around $6 in her bank account due to unexpected situations recently. And she knew that her little boy would be hungry and ask for food once workout was done. I had NO IDEA all that was going on in her life at that time but the Holy Spirit did! His timing is always priceless. My trainer and I were both standing out there crying and were both blessed by God in very different ways. That day God was glorified and my seed was sown into good ground. Over the next several months my weight just melted off. Like really just melted off. I was losing between 10-20 pounds each month but especially inches. During this quick weight loss journey, the Lord gave me wisdom on purchasing clothes. Each month I would buy one pair of black slacks and one pair of gray slacks for work and church. I would buy two or three nice tops and rotate the combinations throughout the week. When those clothes were too big, I would start my process over again- one black, one gray and two or three different tops. Of course, the clothes I really couldn't fit I would sow into the lives of other ladies in need. This process went on until I reached a SIZE 6 in my pants!!!! Praise God!! By December 2014, I had reached my goal and ALL glory, honor and praise goes to God!

Also during this journey, I became a runner. Yes, an actual runner. I love to run now and I truly believe I can run any distance. Well, deep down one of my desires was to run a 5K. I wasn't and hadn't ever trained to run a 5K but I told my trainer about my desire casually in a conversation one day and she informed me about the upcoming Breast Cancer run downtown. I got really excited and signed up almost immediately. The race date came quickly but there was one thing, I had never ran three miles straight before. I figured I should, at least, prepare myself to run three miles straight before the run although I was in good shape. There was a park in town I often walked at that was conveniently three miles long one time around. I usually walk this park on Sundays to wind down and reflect on the week, however, this time at the park I had decided to run as much as I could. I started off walking as a warm up and then said a quick prayer and started running. I ran and kept running to make three miles! That was indeed my very first time running that distance and it felt like there were angels pushing me from behind. I was running, smiling and thanking God that I was actually running! This may sound small to someone else but this was a huge accomplishment for me! The following weekend was the race date. I was really pumped up and focused on this race. I was determined to run the full three miles without stopping. The race began and I led the pack. During my run, I noticed that one of my shoelaces was about to come a loose. OH NO! When I mean I wasn't stopping, I wasn't stopping for anything so I didn't. I said a quick prayer and those shoelaces did not come a loose. I ran my very first 5K in 32 minutes!! I was sooooo excited and still am!

The last thing that my trainer said to me during our conversation that day when my seed was sown into her life was that she was committed to helping me reach my weight loss goal. However, at some point along this journey I realized that the Holy Spirit was transitioning me to have a praying and fasting lifestyle. After the instructed Daniel's Fast was over, maybe a week later, I felt led in my spirit to go on another Daniel's Fast. Month after month, fast after fast, workout after workout the weight literally vanished. The Lord was working a miracle in my body and I was transforming right before my eyes and others. Not only was my body transformed, my mind and spirit was also. Due to the continuous fasting, my spirit was extremely sensitive to the Holy Spirit and my desire for His presence grew almost daily. It is an amazing thing to experience; constant and intentional fellowship with the Holy Spirit. I began to read my Bible more and actually study scriptures to gain more insight and revelation. I also noticed that my prayers were changing. I wasn't constantly praying about my issues and concerns but making a conscious and heartfelt effort to pray on behalf of other people as led by the Holy Spirit. I knew my prayers were making a difference when my Pastor approached me before service one Sunday and said thank YOU for praying for me, I can feel your prayers! I was stunned and really didn't know how to respond. I just said you're welcome. From then on I make sure that I lift up my Pastor and leaders daily. This all happened as a result of my weight loss prayer and God's response to my request!

When I wasn't fasting I made sure to eat lots of veggies! I made a personal decision earlier in my journey to significantly decrease the amount of red meat from my diet. Now, I'm not a vegetarian by any means but I chose chicken and fish as my main protein providers. I also ate brown rice versus white rice and frozen veggies versus the canned veggies. I also doubled my water intake during this journey. Although it becomes extremely annoying to visit the restroom quite often, but this is a clear indicator that your body is hydrated. Another tip was that I ate smaller snacks every two hours or so to increase my metabolism. If you're around me for any length of time you know that I looooove the sweet and salty trail mix that includes fresh roasted peanuts, sunflower kernels, raisins, with a few chocolate M&M's! One more important factor to consider during your weight loss journey is your portion control. Too much of a good thing isn't good for you. This is an area that I must consistently watch.

In the midst of this great experience and journey, I took my focus and determination to another level. At one point, I put my workouts before everything. I worked out religiously. I began enjoying my workout very much plus the results from the workouts manifested almost instantly. It got so bad that I planned my social activities around my workouts. If my friends were interested in going to the movies on a Friday night and the movie started at 7 pm I would insist that we see a later movie because my workouts started at 7 pm. My friends didn't say anything to me that I can remember but I'm SURE they were thinking something was wrong with me. Wanting to workout and intentionally scheduling your workouts in your day isn't a bad thing at all. I had not realized that I had idolized working out until one day as I was leaving my apartment to go workout, I heard the Holy Spirit say, "spend some time with me". WHAT!? Of course, right after my workout, I thought to myself but I KNEW He wanted me to skip workout that day and spend quality time with Him. Wow....what a wake up call! How did this happen? One thing I lacked that I didn't know at the time was the balance. A balance was needed in my prayer life, eating lifestyle and working out. I tell you it all makes a difference. Our God is a jealous God!

"You must worship no other gods, ~~for the~~ LORD, whose very name is Jealous, is a God who is jealous about his relationship with you" Exodus 34:14 NLT

From then on, I made a conscious effort to chill out and truly enjoy this journey. With everything God desires the glory from our lives and He alone deserves it. It was and still is with great excitement that I tell individuals that approached me regarding my journey, that it was ALLLLL God! But they all seem to want more. Therefore, I coined a phrase that I would tell my church family, co-workers, and friends when they inquired, "was that I would pray, eat right and workout…. in that order!"

REFLECTION

I once heard a quote by Cecily Morgan that says, "You're only as good as your word and your word is only as good as your actions". As I reflect on my weight loss journey and write this book to encourage someone, I find myself overwhelmingly grateful to God. Although this journey, like others, is never quite over I thank God almost daily for answering my prayers. It's one thing to believe that God hears your prayers but to have them answered is another thing. But we really shouldn't be shocked or surprised that our prayers are answered if we have an intimate relationship with our Father. That's supposed to happen. Every morning when I enter into the bathroom to get ready for the day, I look in the mirror and simply smile. This journey again was not about me gaining attention but rather me desiring something fresh and new in my life. I had no idea that God would answer my request the way that He did but He is God. This journey is again my personal journey with real-life manifestations. I am by no means promoting a size 6 or any number weight or size for that matter, but I am promoting and encouraging everyone reading these words to Pray (seek God). Eat (healthy). Lift (often) in that order. This combination can and will change your life if actions are taken. I believe it to be God's will for His people to be in good health and prospering

---

"Dear friend, I hope all is well with you and that you are as healthy in body as you are strong in spirit" 3 John 2:2

PRINCIPLES FOR A PRODUCTIVE WEIGHT LOSS JOURNEY

PRINCIPLE 1: Write Your Goals Down

PRINCIPLE 2: Be Consistent

PRINCIPLE 3: No Idolization- Balance

PRINCIPLE 4: Have Fun

PRINCIPLE 5: Remember That It's A Journey

PRINCIPLE 1: Write Your Goals Down

Writing your goals down has a way of making you accountable. It's amazing how your words written on a simple 8-1/2" by 11" piece of paper become your accountability partner. It also helps to review your written goals often especially on those days that you need that extra encouragement because they will come. I strongly recommend that you pray over your goals often as well. And be very specific! One of my friends has mentioned several times after I've prayed with her that I'm very bold and direct with God. I always laugh because I have finally received the revelation that God knows my every thought even before I think it. In this case, why not lay it all on God's altar?

PRINCIPLE 2: Be Consistent

The definition of consistent according to the Merriam-Webster dictionary is always acting or behaving in the same way; of the same quality. Although I got a little carried away at one point during my journey, I remained consistent with the process. I prayed daily and gave thanks in advance for the results, ate better foods, and worked out at least 3 days a week. Some days after a long day at work I didn't even feel like driving to workout but I pressed my way through and I'm glad I did. There will be plenty of things that will come up in your day to take your time and attention away from working out, eating right and even praying. But keeping your written goals in a place that you visit often will not only encourage you but keeps those goals at the front of your mind at all times for consistency.

PRINCIPLE 3: No Idolization- Balance

Please remember to balance your life. Do not worship your

workouts and weight loss like I started to do. Balance is the

answer to this problem. Prioritize your time in each day and be

disciplined to stay on track. Idolization can be a very subtle

process, however, being intentional is necessary.

Oh, you haven't made an idol before? An idol, by simple

definition, is an icon, image, figure or anything that is greatly

admired, loved and worshiped like a god. The Lord clearly states

in the ten commandments to not have any other god but him.

"You must not make for yourself an idol of any kind or an image of anything in the heavens or on the earth or in the sea. You must not bow down to them or worship them, for I, the Lord your God, am a jealous God who will not tolerate your affection for any other gods." Exodus 20:4-5

PRINCIPLE 4: Have Fun

Having fun and enjoying this process is probably the hardest thing to do especially if you hadn't seen the fruit of your hard work yet. I recommend that before you even start your weight loss journey you already believe that you've lost the weight desired. This will eliminate the stress and allows you to relax and have fun. Take my example, I SO believed that this weight was leaving and NEVER returning I gave away my clothes right off the bat! I'm not telling anyone to give away their clothes but do what you have to do to eliminate potential stress along the way. When others see you having fun and enjoying your journey it will indeed encourage them to start their own journey whether you realize it or not.

PRINCIPLE 5: Remember That It's A Journey

Like the quote by Phillip McGraw states, "Life's a marathon, not a sprint". The same concept and attitude should be applied to your weight loss process. Even though I've lost over 70 pounds, that doesn't mean I get to sit around eating pizza and ice cream all day every day. The same habits and lifestyle changes that got me to this point must be maintained for a lifetime. It's a continual journey and learning process. I'm always seeking new ways to eat better and trying new workouts when I'm traveling etc. So know that there are no quick fixes here… it's a life long journey. Therefore, take lots of pictures along the way to track your process and share your journey to those who follow you!

PICTURES

BEFORE PICTURES

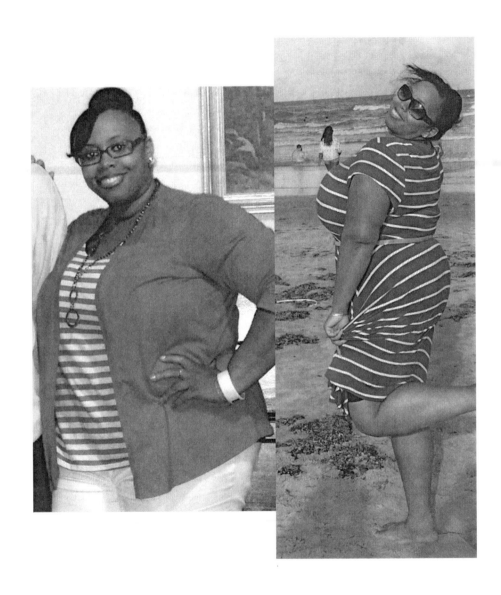

AFTER PICTURES

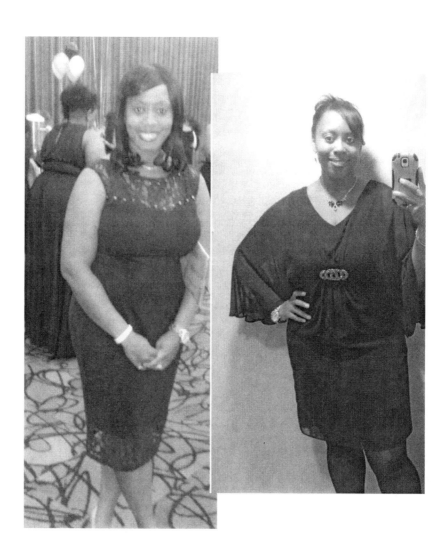

TRANSITION PICTURES

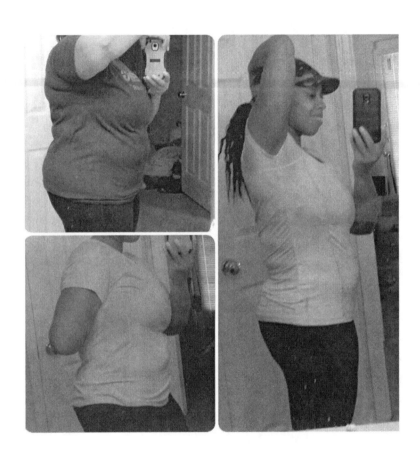

ABOUT THE AUTHOR

As a speaker, author, and entrepreneur, Meagan Pinkney is active in her pursuit to inspire single women on their journey through singleness. Meagan's life is an example to many that your life as a Christian single can be very productive when your time and energy is focused in the right direction. This is the message that Meagan is sharing to women everywhere that she goes. Meagan has earned a Bachelor's degree in Civil Engineering in 2008 from Southern University in Baton Rouge, Louisiana. She earned her MBA in 2012 from Kaplan University as an online student while working full time.

PUBLISHED MATERIAL BY MEAGAN PINKNEY

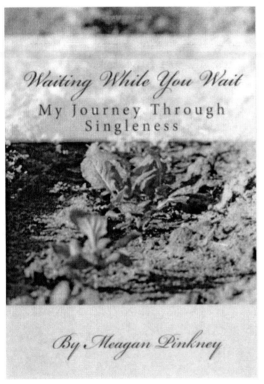

www.waitingwhileyouwait.com

Being a Christian who is single is a tough task in these times due to the tremendous amount of distractions all around. From the pressures of having premarital sex, being a size 0, and being alone on a Friday night (while it is raining and there is nothing on the television while you are snuggled in bed alone...oh sorry.. focus) are just a few things that can affect the productiveness of a single person in the Kingdom of God.

In this book, I will share several personal testimonies from my journey as a single woman as I have learned to wait on God. When a single person yields themself to the Holy Spirit, for the use of the Kingdom, you will be amazed by the testimonies you will be able to share. Instead of me forgetting all the wonderful, supernatural things God has done in and through my life, I wanted to write all of them down to pass on to other single Christians. I believe it is an extremely important task to pass on to others what God can and will do for us if we learn to wait on Him (like a waiter) while we are in the process of waiting (for marriage)! The purpose of this book is to motivate singles to lean on God for everything, whether big or small. God loves us dearly and He wants to see us prosper. Singleness is a beautiful thing and should definitely be valued as it is a blessing from God- whether you are single for a season or a lifetime.

To book Meagan Pinkney or to purchase products and packages please contact her at:

www.meaganpinkney.com
(539) 302-3848

CPSIA information can be obtained
at www.ICGtesting.com
Printed in the USA
FSOW02n0554061216
28199FS